Dealing with Chronic Fibromyalgia Pain with Less Opiates

By Dr. Linda E. Bender

Dealing with Chronic Fibromyalgia Pain with Less Opiates

By Dr. Linda E. Bender

2nd Edition

DISCLAIMER AND TERMS OF USE

Copyright

Most of the content in this book is protected by copyright.

Except as permitted by the copyright law applicable to you, you may not reproduce or communicate any of the content in this book without the permission of the copyright owner.

This may change these terms of use from time to time.

Cover Art

The cover art may not be used without prior written permission.

Disclaimer

The material published in this book is intended for general information only and is not professional advice.

While care and consideration have been taken in the creation of the material in this book, I do not warrant, represent, or guarantee that the material published in this book is in all respects accurate, complete, and current. To the extent permitted by law, we exclude any liability, including any liability for negligence, for any loss or damage arising from reliance on material on this website.

I am not responsible for the content of any third-party website to which links are provided from this website. Any links to websites are provided for your information and convenience only. I do not endorse or control these websites and cannot guarantee that the material on those sites is in all respects accurate, complete, and current.

PROLOG

I am Dr. Linda E. Bender, EdD. EdD is an educational applied doctorate. I am an educator, used to be a college professor in both Anthropology (cultural, physical, and sociolinguistic) and Journalism (mass media and multimedia), and have a tattoo that says there is something more, family is choice, inspire, and teach. That's how much, teaching, and inspiring, are part of my personality and being.

So am I just another self-help author, well yes and no. This is based on self-help but also options of other places to look for help and education of options. There are several routes to dealing with fibromyalgia and chronic pain. When I taught, I taught concepts, not facts and figures. This is what was remembered once the class was over. Facts and figures were forgotten, but the concepts remained. This is how this book is set up. Both will be explained but if one only got the concepts and tried them in a way that worked for them then I would have accomplished something for my fellow sufferers and their support network, "family." Remember family is who has one's back when backed against the wall, and that is offered in reciprocation.

Don't worry, this is not too technical but a first-hand option from a fellow sufferer.

DIAGNOSIS

There is no definitive test for fibromyalgia, it falls in the category of NOS (not otherwise specified) chronic pain. Often it is a lack of other explanations which is why it is so broad.

Mayo Clinic, do a search for fibromyalgia and see what's new. I will summarize This very reputable source here but check it out frequently because they add to and modify it as studies come out.

The overview page explains that fibromyalgia is "widespread musculoskeletal pain accompanied by fatigue, sleep, memory, and mood issues." They also say it can be caused by physical trauma (like with me when I would not listen to an increasingly worse back for over a year and a half till it was pushing on my spinal cord causing weakness in my left leg). It can also be "surgery, infection, or psychological stress." The final catchall is that it can occur over a longer time with no specific trigger.

More likely for women to get it than men.

May also have "tension headaches, TMJ disorders, IBS, anxiety, and depression.

While no cure for fibromyalgia, medications, and "exercise, relation, and stress-reduction measures may help."

My fibromyalgia started two days after my commitment ceremony, when at exactly 39.5 years old I was in the ER with burning and numbness in my groin and genitals and a whacked-out back. Fast forward to a rushed appointment with the back doctor and an MRI. That's when she told me about three bulging disks, one pushing on my spinal cord, but that didn't explain all the pain. I had been in so much pain that before the MRI, the doctor thought we would be doing emergency surgery. Instead, she starts touching places other than my back and numb leg, gets excited, tells me to hold on, comes back with a fibromyalgia brochure, and then has it confirmed by a rheumatologist. After over two years suffering from fibromyalgia, I for sure would have wished for emergency back surgery would have been the ONLY answer. But almost a decade after diagnosis, I am living in the glow of the light at the end of the tunnel level of flair-ups.

SYMPTOMS FOR FIBROMYALGIA INCLUDE:

Widespread pain.

Fatigue (The three days in a row I had fatigue were like having the weakness of a terrible flu.}

Cognitive difficulties "fibro fog".

CAUSES

Causes are unknown but believed to be a combination of genetics, infections, and/or physical or emotional trauma.

The Mayo Clinic's explanation of why it hurts is that; "Researchers believe repeated nerve stimulation causes the brains of people with fibromyalgia to change. This change involves an abnormal increase in levels of certain chemicals in the brain that signal pain (neurotransmitters). In addition, the brain's pain receptors seem to develop a sort of memory of the pain and become more sensitive, meaning they can overact to pain signals."

This brings me to the concept I have developed on the "Pain Train." Once the pain starts in one area, even from a physical injury like hurting an arm, shoulder, hand, back, ankle, etc., the fibromyalgia takes and runs with it adding to it, car by car, by just adding and adding even more links of pain. Now the Mayo Clinic is a great source of information but not the be-all and end-all of it. I have read several books on chronic pain that state that chronic pain rewires one of two pain pathways now through the limbic system, the part of the brain that controls emotion. Therefore, when strong feelings happen, fibromyalgia symptoms may intensify. The stronger the emotion, the more severe the symptoms can be. This typically happens with negative or nonfunctional emotions like anger, frustration, depression, or anxiety, but it can also occur with strong positive emotions such as a promotion or a child's wedding.

WHAT CAN MAKE IT WORSE

There are a few things I have noticed and read about that can make it worse and that is strong (mainly negative} emotions, anxiety, stress, horrible eating, lack of sleep, and a cold. There are several things that can be done to avoid these minefields as much as possible as covered already. But on the cold front, it was a very practical male professional who pointed out that if the cold was an issue, besides the already dressing warmer, get a heating blanket to warm the sheet and work like a full body heating pad when things are getting bad. That uncommon, common sense led to immeciately ordering one. If sharing a bed, a dual zone one is best. Another thing that can irritate a volatile fibromyalgia is not enough sleep. I once had such bad PTSD nightmares I was running out of the house from bed into the garage to feel safer. The first night, this occurred two hours into sleep, and I refused to sleep the rest of the night. The pain was bad but every hour it just increased till 2 pm and I was vomiting from the pain. Then off for an injection of a drug called Toradol so I could sleep.

IMPORTANCE OF SLEEP

There is a paradox with fibromyalgia, harder time sleeping, and less sleep equals more pain. Getting a full night's sleep, and better-quality sleep is even better, is the best way to be as pain-free as possible. Therefore, most fibromyalgia patients are prescribed a sleeping aid. But if not used, good sleep hygiene and things like magnesium or melatonin help get a good night's sleep. Google the first and magnesium and melatonin can be bought over the counter for cheap. Take 5-6 mg of melatonin as a good amount but not more. If suffering the melatonin hangover drops to half. This OTC takes time to accumulate in the system so give it at least 2-6 weeks. Take it at night, most people get an effect in 30 minutes to 2 hours.

TREATMENTS

Treatments I use daily are diversion/distraction, deep breathing, medications (strong non-inflammatory, Neurontin [also known as gabapentin, etc.], watching what I eat, and staying warm. Treatments I use several times a week include Tylenol, lidocaine cream, massage, and heat. Weekly can include gym, aqua therapy, hot tub, chiropractic care, acupuncture, or physical therapy massage. Less than that is: sleeping pills, Toradol, and as a last resort, an opiate pill.

PAIN MANAGEMENT PROGRAMS

Many insurances cover, even recommend, pain management programs for chronic pain sufferers just to keep down opiate use. In the old days that meant they dispensed the drugs. But that has changed, and the reason is because of a woman I met and many more like her. She has fibromyalgia and 12 years ago went to the health insurance "pain management" program. Fast forward 12 years later, I met her. She was using a walker (but also older) I was wheelchair-bound beyond 100 feet, and she proudly announced, even advertised she was on Fentanyl patches. She was heading off to get one of her 3 times weekly morphine injections. Well medically other than morphine drips this lady was maxed out and was in her 60s. There was little space left to go, she was an addict. She was telling a group of people how painful fibromyalgia was but there was no wincing, bent over, erratic posture, or walking. This is where the opiate epidemic came from, heading off the pain rather than treating it.

When joining a new thinking pain management program there is a pain management doctor who controls the pain medication at the lowest level and keeps trying to lower the levels of narcotics so that addiction is less likely to occur. In fact, on the intake questionnaire, there will be several questions asking if one takes the medication because it has been 4-6 hours to prevent pain or because there is pain, and it is not scheduled. The best position to be in is the latter. That is why the current thinking is to prescribe 10-15 opiates a month instead of daily or multiple times a day. In California where I live, addictive meds can only be prescribed short term through an ER or longer term (chronic) through the primary doctor or pain management doctor and there is drug screening every 6 months to make sure to catch abuse, the consequence of abusing opiates or other drugs (street) is the immediate stopping of the prescriptions. In fact, in California legalized medicinal marijuana has been legal for about a decade and recently legal for anyone over 21.

Pain management is playing a larger and larger role in the prescribed opiates and such because of these crackdowns that are not just California but a national crisis. So, pain management is often to the benefit of not just fibromyalgia but any chronic pain. This is where one learns tools to reach for before the prescription bottle(s). Then there is a Pain psychologist and/or Marriage and Family Therapist (MFT) and often a pain RN. The point is to work on all aspects of chronic pain, with a more holistic focus. This way of looking at multiple facets allows for not only the medication aspects but also physical therapy, counseling, being taught Cognitive Behavioral Therapy (CBT) and Dialectical Behavioral Therapy (DBT) to deal with challenges, depression, frustration, anger, anxiety, fear, etc., plus often they let the client bring a guest, which is often the caretaker and discuss the pull upon them. A big part of these types of programs is to break down and give reinforcement for the "baby steps" process of learning to regain what one had before chronic pain.

There is also a physical therapist that helps regain movement and function. For me, since hurting my back and fibromyalgia occurring at the same time I am really limited in walking. There is pain in the lower back, quick numbness, and lack of stability but also due to the "Pain Train" the back pain always triggers fibromyalgia in at least both thighs if not the upper body. So, walking with cramped thighs led to hunching over in walking, irritating the back, which further irritated the fibromyalgia in the thighs. This led to over 6 months of traveling via wheelchair to help the back relax and heal without further annoying it (and me). But due to this, my core muscles got weak, and so did my back and thighs. So, PT was more stretches and using the body as resistance to help. Every person with fibromyalgia has different symptoms, leading to complexity in diagnoses which can be done by any of numerous doctors, one's primary or any specialty doctor (mine was a back doctor) but often one will be sent to a Rheumatologist for confirmation since this is their area of specialty.

WHO CAN OFFICIALLY DIAGNOSE

I was originally told that I probably had this horrible pain due to fibromyalgia by a back doctor, but a Rheumatologist gave me an official diagnosis, but a primary doctor, any medical doctor, or a psychiatrist can make the final call. No matter who one hears it from there is a double-edged sword of, "I'm not crazy and imagining this" and "Oh, no, please be wrong." Followed by what caused this, what is this, what can I expect, and is there a cure? If not, what is the treatment? The last is a basic "Oh no" or "Oh wow."

Fibromyalgia is like the waves that ebb and flow, waves can be higher, lower, riptides, crest, long periods between, or even still water for a while. But like the surf, there will always be changes, maybe by a few minutes, hours, or a day or two. The techniques in this book will help teach one to "surf" through the cresting waters and just sit on the board between waves enjoying the peace and quiet, but prepared for the next swell, for unfortunately, it will just be a matter of time.

Rheumatologist

Often fibromyalgia is added as a diagnosis from a rheumatologist, who can prescribe things like a fitting exercise, lidocaine cream, non-inflammatory, something to deal with the overactive nerves like Neurontin, Lyrica, etc., and an anti-depressant because with chronic illness, especially pain, depression is almost a given, unfortunately. Since I was already diagnosed with bipolar and PTSD, I was already on Neurontin and an anti-depressant, they just had to be adjusted. Don't be surprised if the anti-depressant on the doctor's first try is Cymbalta because it is known to also help with the pain. But I got side effects and had to change back. So, remember it takes 4-8 weeks to fully find out how a medication is going to work and if exploring the scientific method, one variable (medication) at a time.

Psychiatrist

No one is "crazy" and "imagining" the symptoms but there is a belief that chronic pain re-routes (miss-wire) through the limbic system. A small little kidney bean-sized area of the brain where the emotions are handled. That is why strong (especially negative) emotions can cause instant cramping or other symptoms. I already had one and like I said I was already on two drugs used for it that only had to be increased. But also, through this doctor, I found I could take a half dosage of a sleeping aid aimed at "cooling" an overactive limbic system. And if it came back or I needed to cut the day short I took the other half. But never two days in a row. At the worst, I averaged 5-7 or so halves, with 2-3 days being a full dosage in pieces.

Since the limbic can be involved then counseling in Cognitive Behavioral Therapy (CBT) and/or Dialectical Behavioral Therapy (DBT) can be used to deal with challenges, depression, frustration, anger, anxiety, fear, etc. These options can be beneficial, plus often there are caretaker issues, and this can be discussed as the issue of always pulling upon the caretaker(s). CBT is great for understanding things like distorted (or stinking) thinking. This concept is broken into many areas but the main one I found myself doing because of fibromyalgia was overgeneralizing and future telling, I'm in pain, I always will be. I am limited, I will always be. The reality is once I started reading and researching, I made the bulk of it go away for short to long periods of time. Sometimes the worst missed me for, at first a day, then days, weeks, or eventually most of months at a time. I have setbacks I can't control, like cold and the weather, but the parts that hit through the limbic system I could. Another distortion was the should have, would have, and could have. A very seasoned psychologist taught me how this works and he stated for us to remember it as "you should on yourself, you Sh*t on yourself." This is true, I used it with I should have gotten better by now, I should be able to do more for myself, In the past I could have. I would love for this to all go away. Don't defecate on oneself, I had to remind myself.

DBT teaches how to stay in the moment. Yes, I too wanted to escape any "moment" the fibromyalgia was bad, but I used DBT's mindfulness to focus on the present. Yes, the present had a lot of pain, but while my thighs were cramping, etc., I could focus on an object: its size, design, cool touch, smell, weight, what it sounds like when I tap it, etc. This makes me focus on that instead of the pain. By doing that well, I would derail any more cars of the "Pain Train" if not my ribs would tighten up next. Pain is a great reason to learn lessons faster. I was highly motivated to get as far to the other side of the pain as I could.

The emotions of depression, frustration, anger, anxiety, fear, etc., would just overheat the limbic, and the "Pain Train" would roll out and the stronger the emotions the faster the "cars" were added. The result was me curled in a ball crying from my whole-body clench, and my skin feeling like it was being cut in crisscross patterns all over my body. As I learned to put emotions in the concept of an emotion is just an emotion, I can have emotions but need to make sure they don't "have" me. I was angry over PTSD stuff and frustrated and anxious about the pain. When I didn't use this concept (which I read in a CBT book for a pain management program) The pain just got worse and worse till I was curled in a ball. At pain management, I learned my new 10 was curled in a ball past the 911 call. With fibromyalgia, one can have tons of those moments.

With unresolved emotional issues (mainly PTSD), I was getting nailed by strong, negative emotions. I learned quickly to put as many of my strong emotions that were mainly negative in a box. An emotion is an emotion. My past sucked, I don't want to forgive or forget, but I need to not focus strongly on it or let it overwhelm me, otherwise, I pay with serious pain, not any of "those" people.

So, between tools in my toolbox ranging from CBT's tricks and those of DBT both of which overlap on meditation and deep breathing as calming skills, I was able to derail adding cars or even letting the "Pain Train" get up to full speed. The tracks will forever be there because I have fibromyalgia and with a disorder with no concretely known causes, and no definitive test for it, it will be a while before there can be a cure or way of reversing it. But I can slow the "Pain Train" and keep down the number of "cars" it has.

DIET AND EXERCISE

Diet

There are several suggestions on diet. I have heard of the wonders of the Paleolithic diet. All the vegetables, grain, and meats of early man which means: no milk, eggs, chicken, beef, or pork. Or even plant-based diets (vegan}. I couldn't do it but as I incorporated the mayo diet recipes in my food for dinner and sometimes lunch the pain reduced so there is some truth there. But I couldn't do more than several substitutions but don't hesitate to try it. The healthier you are the less it will bother you. Some people just take out gluten, eggs, and/or milk and find some relief.

Experiment with your food choices. See if they are worth the time, money, and sacrifice. Remember it will take about two weeks to see the results. Scientific method says the best tests are changing one variable at a time to see what the key variable is. When doing this keep a food log that logs meals and snacks and the pain to see how they are connected that day and the next two or three days.

Healthy eating will make you feel better. That is guaranteed, but the benefit is that the reduced weight will stress the body less and remember that gets rid of cars on the "Pain Train". Just a concept. If wondering what cookbook, a way would be to try to eat more of a Paleolithic diet but still taste good and have some "normal" in average grocery store ingredients, try the cookbook Fix-It and Enjoy -IT Healthy Cookbook by Phyllis Pellman Good with nutritional expertise from Mayo clinic. They coordinated with the Mayo Clinic food pyramid which is based on this concept. There is an educational section, and it is well broken into segments. The writer taste tested before just going "Oh, look, healthy stuff, then mix it together for a healthy meal that tastes like tree bark." I found that 3 days on this diet a week reduced the fibromyalgia flair-ups and daily pain by about 80%.

Exercise

These next two forms of exercise are suggested by many doctors to fibromyalgia sufferers, yoga, and aqua aerobics/therapy because they are low impact and will often help way more than hurt. There is also the gym and at minimum the exercises of a physical therapist.

These next two forms of exercise are suggested by many doctors to fibromyalgia sufferers, yoga, and aqua aerobics/therapy because they are low impact and will often help way more than hurt. There is also the gym and at minimum the exercises of a physical therapist.

Yoga – I want to admit I had done this on a few occasions pre-fibromyalgia and with a not-so-great back. I tried about 5 different times in the span of a few months and by the 4th time, I had the same instructor as the last time I went. The reason I quit was she was the main one at my gym and my back being always not so perfect I was never able to be as flexible with it. On that fateful fifth session, she kept telling me to get lower and I said I couldn't, and she came over to prove I could by pushing on my lower back and hurting me in the process. So, there is caution in finding the right teacher/instructor. That was over a decade ago before the invasiveness of YouTube and all their free yoga clips. There are also inexpensive DVDs besides the more expensive classes.

The concept is to stretch, strengthen, and center your mind and body. All of this is great for fibromyalgia. It's easy to try at home for a cheap beach towel or $15 yoga mat, some space, preferably a mirror to check your position in. It slowly stretches muscles with your own body and gravity doing the work and boy can it work up a sweat, even a version called chair yoga, an even lower impact of yoga.

One of the problems with fibromyalgia is that muscles, tendons, ligaments, skin, nerves misfire, and conduct errors often in the form of muscle or constricting and hurting like you just ran a marathon or was pounding weights for the first time in the gym. Yoga loosens those muscles and increases blood flow to parts of the body including the brain re-centering part. It also increases serotonin and that helps with depression and chronic illnesses will cause depression, like chronic pain. Plus, it cools off the limbic system making you feel more centered in your world and decreasing the intensity of strong emotions that can activate fibromyalgia.

Need more motivation than watching a video at home, trying apps on the phone, or signing up for classes letting the instructor know you have limitations. The goal is to work past them but remember that these limitations change not only day by day and week by week, but also by minute. For those who need it, there is chair yoga.

Water exercise – Years ago, I went to several water yoga classes at gyms because it was a great way for a full body, cardiovascular workout with arthritic, post-operative knees. My overall experience was the classes were made of older, heavier, and less overall in shape people who saw a way to get a good workout with less impact. The water is not only for buoyancy but also resistance to moving and that is the benefit.

Now I have a bad back with weight put on from being basically in a wheelchair body for over 6 months while on high steroids for the back and then asthma issue and putting on 60 pounds in just over 6 months. Making everything hurt even more. But the back surgeon said I had to lose 80 pounds before I could have surgery to fix the fact that my leg went numb within minutes of standing/walking on it. She said she told her patients who had any weight issues and many who didn't walk laps in the pool. Low-impact muscle building. I tried the association-heated outdoor pool and could go 3 times further in water up to my breasts, dragging on my arms, doing high knee walks, or pretending I was, then I would hit the hot tub for 5-10 minutes and do another lap or two the same way. It worked excellently and one day doing about a mile total in walking in segments, I was significantly free of most of the daily pain for up to two additional days. I met on vacation a woman from Tennessee who had a bad back and fibromyalgia and tried just standard water aerobics in the pool and ended up more sore. Again, outdoor backyard pool and too much out-of-water aerobics part. She liked the idea of walking and trying to run in mid-chest deep water.

Gym – I have been a competitive athlete for over a decade, so I love working out in the gym and have done this not only with professional personal trainers but also with semi-professional bodybuilders who were competitive in the field and loved hitting the weights. But stretching is better than the strength for fibromyalgia daily. But I have learned that going to the gym is great, but some precautions should be taken. One, have a driver in case there is fibromyalgia tightening of the leg muscles or arm muscles creating an unsafe driving situation. Also, look for a gym with hydro massage machines available for free with your membership a hot tub or both. These make it ok most of the time to go solo if used at the end of a workout to relax the muscles needed for driving. When doing weightlifting circuits try a low number of repetitions like 5-10 and do those repetitions twice before moving on. Keep the weight low but know that if all goes well one can cycle back through again. This avoids the "Pain Train".

I want to admit I had done this on a few occasions pre-fibromyalgia and with a not-so-great back. I tried about 5 different times in the span of a few months and by the 4th time, I had the same instructor as the last time I went. The reason I quit was she was the main one at my gym and my back being always not so perfect I was never able to be as flexible with it. On that fateful fifth session, she kept telling me to get lower and I said I couldn't, and she came over to prove I could by pushing on my lower back and hurting me in the process. So, there is caution in finding the right teacher/instructor. That was over a decade ago before the invasiveness of YouTube and all their free yoga clips. There are also inexpensive DVDs besides the more expensive classes.

The concept is to stretch, strengthen, and center your mind and body. All of this is great for fibromyalgia. It's easy to try at home for a cheap beach towel or $15 yoga mat, some space, preferably a mirror to check your position in. It slowly stretches muscles with your own body and gravity doing the work and boy can it work up a sweat, even a version called chair yoga, an even lower impact of yoga.

One of the problems with fibromyalgia is that muscles, tendons, ligaments, skin, nerves misfire, and conduct errors often in the form of muscle or constricting and hurting like you just ran a marathon or was pounding weights for the first time in the gym. Yoga loosens those muscles and increases blood flow to parts of the body including the brain re-centering part. It also increases serotonin and that helps with depression and chronic illnesses will cause depression, like chronic pain. Plus, it cools off the limbic system making you feel more centered in your world and decreasing the intensity of strong emotions that can activate fibromyalgia.

Need more motivation than watching a video at home, trying apps on the phone, or signing up for classes letting the instructor know you have limitations. The goal is to work past them but remember that these limitations change not only day by day and week by week, but also by minute. For those who need it, there is chair yoga.

Water exercise – Years ago, I went to several water yoga classes at gyms because it was a great way for a full body, cardiovascular workout with arthritic, post-operative knees. My overall experience was the classes were made of older, heavier, and less overall in shape people who saw a way to get a good workout with less impact. The water is not only for buoyancy but also resistance to moving and that is the benefit.

Now I have a bad back with weight put on from being basically in a wheelchair body for over 6 months while on high steroids for the back and then asthma issue and putting on 60 pounds in just over 6 months. Making everything hurt even more. But the back surgeon said I had to lose 80 pounds before I could have surgery to fix the fact that my leg went numb within minutes of standing/walking on it. She said she told her patients who had any weight issues and many who didn't walk laps in the pool. Low-impact muscle building. I tried the association-heated outdoor pool and could go 3 times further in water up to my breasts, dragging on my arms, doing high knee walks, or pretending I was, then I would hit the hot tub for 5-10 minutes and do another lap or two the same way. It worked excellently and one day doing about a mile total in walking in segments, I was significantly free of most of the daily pain for up to two additional days. I met on vacation a woman from Tennessee who had a bad back and fibromyalgia and tried just standard water aerobics in the pool and ended up more sore. Again, outdoor backyard pool and too much out-of-water aerobics part. She liked the idea of walking and trying to run in mid-chest deep water.

Gym – I have been a competitive athlete for over a decade, so I love working out in the gym and have done this not only with professional personal trainers but also with semi-professional bodybuilders who were competitive in the field and loved hitting the weights. But stretching is better than the strength for fibromyalgia daily. But I have learned that going to the gym is great, but some precautions should be taken. One, have a driver in case there is fibromyalgia tightening of the leg muscles or arm muscles creating an unsafe driving situation. Also, look for a gym with hydro massage machines available for free with your membership a hot tub or both. These make it ok most of the time to go solo if used at the end of a workout to relax the muscles needed for driving. When doing weightlifting circuits try a low number of repetitions like 5-10 and do those repetitions twice before moving on. Keep the weight low but know that if all goes well one can cycle back through again. This avoids the "Pain Train".

HOLISTIC MEDICINE

Physical therapy

This helps with stretching the muscles, plus with gaining back any weakness caused by avoiding using, the more likely to tighten areas. Remember that any good physical therapist will allow for the exercise to be put in smaller repetitions if the fibromyalgia starts being active. One bad day does not mean throwing out the whole concept forever.

Chiropractic care

A good chiropractor is one that is NOT a bone popper. They are the ones that massage most of the time and pop only a little. This helps because as the body tenses, the biomechanical alignment of the body (hips, legs, back, neck, shoulders) gets out of alignment and can cause long-term damage if not accounted for. Most insurance will cover this, at least in part. I have had my back so tense that I have felt it pop my spine out of alignment. Besides, this again goes to the "Pain Train" theory that if out of alignment there will be biomechanical pain that will only be added to by the pain activating the fibromyalgia which creates even more problems.

Physical Therapy Massages

I paid out of pocket weekly when the fibromyalgia was horrible daily. Physical therapy massage is done not for pampering but when having fibromyalgia, a survival technique. What I found at my place was at the time, there were three technicians. Like Goldilocks of the fairytale, one worked great when in a fibromyalgia crawling ball, but she left me sore for a different reason for almost as long as the benefits were a little too rough. The second worked, and the gentle hands felt good. However, the benefits were short-lived and too soft. The third time I tried was in the middle and worked out the knots, but I was only sore for half an hour or so and got a few days of relief from the 10s on the pain scale. Finding one that works takes some trial and error.

What I learned from this is that whoever massages out the knots should work from outside in to keep down re-knotting. From outside ribs to the spine, one knot at a time. Also, I have found a liniment to help, a rollerball best, and if ready to hit someone trying to help, add a layer of lidocaine cream and let it dry thoroughly before trying liniment and massage if at home.

Acupuncture

This is a new thing for me but seems successful so far. The one I go to is Mike with a double Masters, one in oriental medicine. He told me up front several things. One, it can cause a minor flare if not already flared. I was, so I was not worried. Two, the first treatment only lasts a few hours, but there is a culminating effect that takes 6-12 sessions to achieve. The first time I went in, in the late afternoon I had been threatening to kill people if they were so much as touched me. I was in so much pain and so sensitive. After the session, I went from a deadly level of pain (a 9) to a manageable level (a 5). I could feel the pain, but it wasn't unbearable, and I was able to walk upright. This relief lasted for over three hours and continued until I went to bed (at a pain level of 8). The following two weeks were significantly better than the previous few days. This pattern continued for the next four sessions, resulting in weeks of relief.

MEDICATIONS

There are several options for medications and levels of usefulness. Remember, the pain scale goes from 0 – no pain to 10 – curled in a ball crying and past calling 911. There are several options before opiates which may not get rid of all the pain, but even if it does, it is only for 4-6 Hours. Often less than that, but that's the most it will work. If I were to take them, it only worked for a few hours. If I were to take them preemptory, I would be highly likely to be one of countless opiate addicts. I would rather have words like cranky and touchy used about me than words like addicted and dependent.

What I have tried and how it worked for me on the above pain skill is listed below from lowest to highest.

Tylenol will help bring it down one level, two at best, but if I am just at a 6, I try it. A 1 to 4 I can ignore, 5 is where I am aware of it, and 6 is where I start to try things.

Muscle rubs (liniments, over the counter or homeopathic) This helps with a tightening of muscles and will take it down at least 2 points. The key is that the ingredients be menthol/Eucalyptus. These both provide relief and increase blood flow in the area. At more than 2 points above baseline, this can be painful to rub/massage. A rollerball helps.

Lidocaine creams (over the counter or prescribed) will numb the area, and since it is topical it helps the nerves and muscles relax. If more than 2 points above baseline, try to use this cream, letting it dry, then try a muscle rub/massage with muscle cream. The key is to wait about 5 minutes between applications of each.

NSAIDs

Ibuprofen will help with the inflammation of the muscles and nerves by several points but when using NSAIDs there is a maximum number in 24 hours one should take. NSAIDs can cause gastrointestinal bleeds if one takes too much in a day or consistently.

Mobic is stronger than Ibuprofen, but also an NSAID so when taking it (daily prescription) don't take regular Ibuprofen or other NSAIDs. This is a great help to me to lower my baseline. When taken off Mobic for several days, I ended up curled in a ball then we figured out that this change was causing it and again, put me on it.

Toradol is an even stronger NSAID that is an injection. I have a standing order for up to two a month of a double dose. This will help me go from a 9 to a 4 or below. However, I must not take any other NSAID for 24 hours because it is such a high level of NSAID. But there is a secret to this, if I go to urgent care or ER and tell them I need something for fibromyalgia and that Toradol is what I am seeking (not opiates) I usually get in fast and get out in under 2 hours, pain reduced to next to nothing or nothing.

Neurontin is a prescription used commonly for nerve issues. It works well at low doses and can go quite high in dosage so there is plenty of room to find the right dosage. It has plenty of generics, the most common is Gabapentin. This drug is based on the neurotransmitter GABA, the same neurotransmitter of alcohol except it has no other issues and is not physically addictive. Think of how people on alcohol can bump into things or stumble and not feel a thing until the next day. It slows the nerves and therefore muscle activity. It works great. An increased dosage allowed me to not have to wear pants with thermal underclothes during southern California winters averaging 50s, 60s, and low 70s. WARNING: When starting or doing dosage increases it is best to watch driving, possibly even walking far. Since it is like alcohol it will probably (if taken at night) help with sleep. Less sleep = more pain.

Cymbalta (an anti-depressant) is the most commonly prescribed anti-depressant since it also works to help with the pain. But if not on this anti-depressant, any other will still help with the blues of a chronic, very painful disorder. Remember, strong emotions (especially negative ones) can increase the level of pain one feels.

TV Commercial Medications – I'll be honest, I haven't tried these, but I have done that by choice. I didn't like some of the possible side-effects which on one was early onset dementia. So read labels and warnings carefully and decide if the plus is bigger than the potential minuses.

Sleeping pills can help get that nightly, needed sleep but be careful, most can be addictive. If told not to take one more than every 2-3 nights, then it is probably addictive, and follow the doctor's orders carefully. Don't hesitate to ask for possibly getting a prescription because sometimes the pain can keep one awake, and the pain the next day is even worse. Melatonin is a safe alternative that is over the counter. It can be found anywhere that supplements are sold. The key is to not exceed 5-6 mg as beyond this is not beneficial for sleep but can increase something called by users a melatonin hangover. This can last from an hour to all day. To work best, this drug should be taken within an hour of planned sleeping time and should be taken daily.

Opiates – There is an escalating spectrum of opiates. If needed, take the lowest prescription that helps, and NEVER take them on a planned schedule (such as every 4-6 hours) such as 8 am, noon, 4 pm, 8 pm). Take them ONLY as needed if it is not too early from the last dose. Try not to take them daily. There are plenty of other options before escalating to opiates. Try them, and at different pain points. Some things work better than others.

MANAGE PAIN OR IT MANAGES YOU

If I don't manage the pain then I get knocked down by the "Pain Train" and am left a painful corpse, not able to function or enjoy life. When first diagnosed, with the back issue also, I was left being functional for 15 minutes to 30-45 minutes of ice, heat, massage chair, etc. It was horrible and lifeless. That reality made me depressed and angry. This was before I developed the capability to just say and feel that an emotion was just an emotion, so I was more and more thrashed as the hours went by.

It bothered me that I had no life and every third day I went to the ER for toroidal. I was a 10 or 11 on the fibromyalgia scale, curled in a ball crying, long past most ER trips or 911. I had the distorted thought that I would always be curled up in pain. This was the new baseline. A good day was a 7, the lowest number of the day. But what I found, as I did bibliotherapy, as a doctorate holder and educator I read many books, most were good, and a few were a waste of money. That this was largely a mind game, head over body (and pain). After I had practiced technique after technique, most with success, I had a baseline that dropped to a 5-6 after 6-9 months. After 9-12 months, I had a baseline of 4-5. That baseline I could ignore most of the day.

Most people would be at least going to the doctor, if not urgent care/ER if they didn't have fibromyalgia. Sorry, a baseline means, for me, some stiffness/tightness every day, but most of the time I can ignore it. It has become less and less every 3-6 months as I get better and better at using these techniques.

After 10 years, I am down to occasional flair-ups. This is due to not only the techniques in this book but also the treatment of the original spinal issues bothering me and therapy to help with the pain-train from emotional issues.

Try, Try, Try

The one thing that kept me searching and may lead others to read is the search for a richer life to feel more like one is fully alive, or at least as much as possible. I refused to allow fibromyalgia to fully take away my quality of life. If this means getting a caretaker like I have, it does. There are government programs for those on Medicaid or some on Medicare. The caretaker does not have to be a spouse or even a relative. In fact, if one needs it and knows no one they have a list of providers.

Caretakers

The role of caretaker can be challenging or even cause depression and frustration. As the recipient, being in chronic pain, I know I could get demanding and sharp because of my frustration and pain so it is possible and common. There are caregiver support groups and as a recipient, it is important to always consider the other person does not have to help even if they love you. Often, especially if the one caretaker did/does ask about how you're feeling or what can they do to help, the chronic pain sufferers need to remember to ask how the caretaker is doing. Plus, remember they have their own lives and thoughts because sometimes, chronic sufferers get in the habit of just talking about how they are suffering and forgetting the first part mentioned. I know I did, and my wife started to feel caretaker mainly/first and wife second/last.

Bibliotherapy

What a great sounding word is "Bibliotherapy" which means things like informational and self-help books. I do that when there is a new issue with me, and I (always) want to take the least amount of pills. I KNOW the brain is so powerful and have seen it help me overcome a lot of issues or at least make them more bite-sized and manageable.

So, the first book I suggest reading is from a doctor named Daniel G. Amen and his wonderful book, "Change Your Brain, Change Your Life".

"The Fix-It and Enjoy-It Healthy Cookbook" by Phyllis Pellman Good with nutritional expertise from Mayo Clinic. 400 great recipes that taste good and balance the line of the Paleolithic food pyramid.

A clinician's book on setting up and running a pain management program can help with exercises one would get from a pain management book called, "CBT for Chronic Pain and Psychological Well Being: A Skills Training Manual Integrating DBT, ABT, Behavior Activation and Motivational Interviewing".

Another CBT/DBT book to read to learn these techniques at a more common language level is "Heal Your Emotions: A Practical Guide to Speaking Your Brain's Languages and Turning Pain into Power" by Shaun Roundy.

The last book comes with a warning, I didn't (fully) agree with it. "The Mind Body Prescription: Healing the Body, Healing the Pain" by Dr. John E. Sarno. This was a book I heard of from someone who had gone through the pain management classes ahead of me. I needed help NOW! Before waiting for the next sessions to start, Dr. Sarno explains how anger can cause many disorders and illnesses (including fibromyalgia). This book is good for how it breaks down pain in the brain, but I thought in my first few weeks of fibromyalgia that anger, ALONE, could not be causing this pain. When I got over the issues I had with people for why my back got hurt, setting off the fibromyalgia, the daily intensity dropped significantly. Doctors had said, "Why don't you forgive these people?" I replied, "They are still alive". He let it drop. What helped is that by holding onto being angry with them I was just hurting myself. I didn't have to forgive or forget, just not dwell in strong negative emotions. But even when the anger was set aside, I still hurt badly, just not constantly horrific.

STRESS

In the world we live in, it is impossible to eliminate stress completely, but we can reduce it, and we can reframe it. What if instead of saying being stressed by a report that was dropped on my desk for a rush turnaround, I saw this as a challenge, would do my best, and that would be all that is possible.

I reduce my access to the news when I'm very symptomatic. Turn off Facebook near bedtime. Go in the hot tub or take a bath. Maybe try some stretches.

If my ribs are tight and I am having trouble breathing, I have two options: freak and stress out or relax and cope. The best thing I have found to do is to breathe as deep and slowly as possible pain permitted till the pain lessens. Not a quick fix but takes 5-10 minutes. CBT has something called Brain Math where I cross my arms over my chest and think of a particularly happy time that brings a huge smile to my face. Then once I had the image, I breathed in over a steady 4 seconds and repeated on out. Repeating frequently until I was happy and relaxed. This took 5-10 minutes the first time and now, years later, I often go to bed doing this and it takes under a minute, and I don't have to hug myself, just imagine and breathe.

As I was writing this, we had a water leak in the slab of our house where pipes had to be rerouted causing holes in drywall that had to have a contractor come in to fix. We were given 3 days' notice to clear the room. We were scheduled for a movie, so we went, and I felt like there was something in my chest cutting the muscle inside connected to the rib cage and pulling these strips apart. As we worked on the house and some progress was made, this pain was left for the final time.

CONCLUSION

This is a very real disorder, not a figment of imagination, an excuse, or hypochondria. It hurts, sometimes unbearably, and sometimes it is hardly noticeable. It needs to be treated as a chronic issue. Even if one does not necessarily feel it one day, it is still there like coach roaches hiding from the light. Eventually, the lights go out, and it's their world again. These are some things that can be used as philosophies or outlooks, or treatment plans to reduce the impulse to first grab the opiates to cover the pain. The best, longest lasting treatments are healthy living and acupuncture. I know neither of those may sound good, but that is the best track I have found. I am not a health nut, but I have lived the southern California food choices for decades, and I used to be an athlete. Although, a COMPLETE, pure, healthy life, I do not always succeed. There is a spectrum from living a long relatively pain-free life and enjoying life. Somewhere between is where most people live. No caffeine, processed sugar, nicotine, and lots of sleep will all lead to a large reduction of pain but that for most, including me, leads to large sacrifices. Balance needs to be arrived so that one is aware that some things won't help the fibromyalgia but will give others solace.

I have read much and tried much, both physically and mentally, a life with less overly strong negative emotion will help too. This is a subject we must use bibliotherapy (like this book) and trial and error to see what works. Learn what you can from many sources of all the options at one's discretion. The main thing one can do is search for one's own truth on this subject, and really any other, and use as many options as possible before popping that magic pill, especially on a preventative schedule.